I0116771

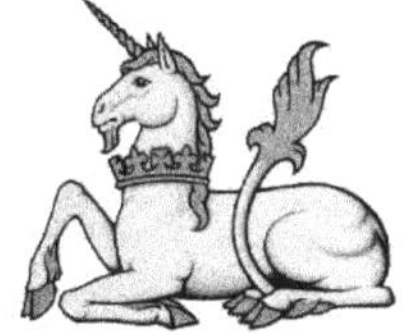

To all who suffer

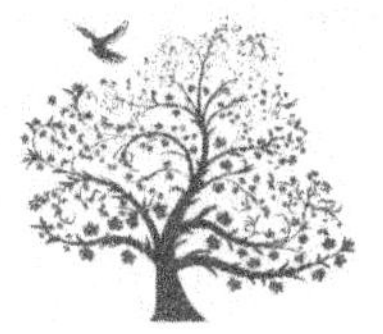

“Homeopathy in Practice”
by Dr. Mirjana Zivanov

Translator:
Dr. Andreas Kelemen

Design and layout:
Dr. Andreas Kelemen

Printed by Create Space

ISBN: 978-86-914263-2-3

Visit our web site at www.homeopathyinpractice.org

CIP - Katalogizacija u publikaciji
Biblioteka Matice srpske, Novi Sad
615.015.32

Zivanov, Mirjana
Homeopathy in Practice/ Zivanov Mirjana; [translated by Andreas Kelemen] - Novi Sad : M. Zivanov, 2012 (USA : Create Space).- 140 str. : ilustr. ; 22 cm
Izv. stv. nasl.: Homeopatska medicina-terapija

ISBN 978-86-914263-2-3
a) Homeopatija
COBISS.SR-ID 269676807

Dr. Mirjana Zivanov

Homeopathy in Practice

Novi Sad
2012

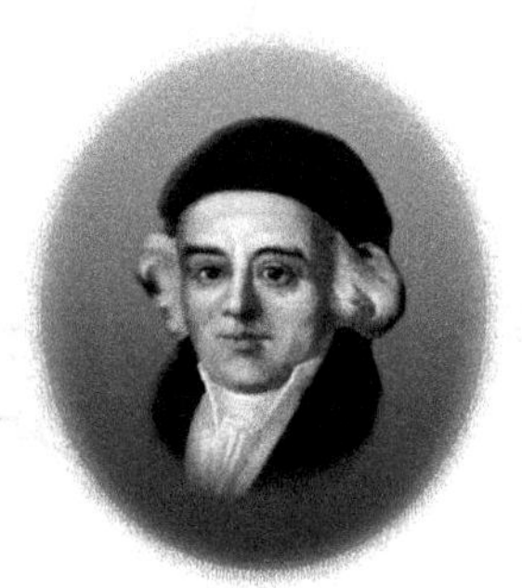

Contents

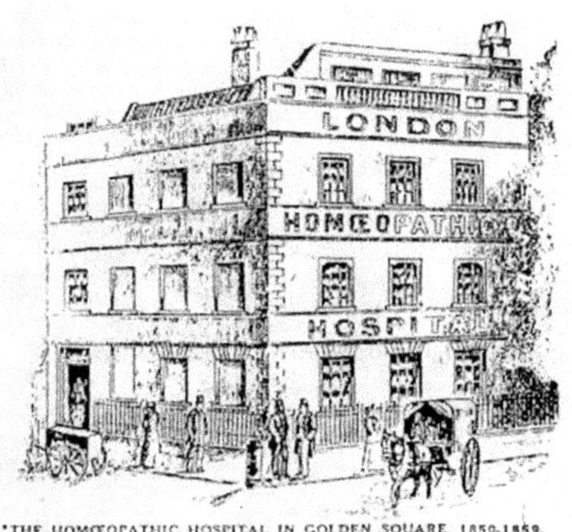

*THE HOMŒOPATHIC HOSPITAL IN GOLDEN SQUARE, 1850-1859.
25 Beds.

Introduction

Homeopathy on health and lifestyle

We wish to introduce people to the homeopathic medicine, the medicine of today and tomorrow. Homeopathy is a branch of the holistic medicine, the medicine that observes a man as a whole, the way he really is – impartial, complete and unique.

We want to show that homeopathic practice is more than successful in treating any kind of disease, or better – disorder. Because the disease is nothing more than a state in which a man is in.

This is a state which is created and exists, but which is always possible to change.

During homeopathic treatment a man leaves this altered state and gets back to his optimal state, his own vibration, so to say, in which he lives in full consciousness, health and freedom. He is free in a sense that he can make the right choices, The ones that will lead him to maturing of both consciousness and spirit.

There are numerous reasons which may disrupt a person's ideal vibration, his own Golden ratio. With the fast development of modern civilization. There is an ever increasing number of factors that can disrupt the order and tranquility in the human soul. This order and tranquility we should always cherish is our ideal vibration, the one that heals us and knows what's best for us. It may be felt most intensely in our heart, so let's listen to our hearts – It whispers the truth.

After a successful homeopathic treatment a patient returns in the state of health in which he used to be, when he was in peace with himself and others. When in this state, he has a chance to preserve it with a new healthy lifestyle. Man in such a state does good deeds to people around him, to children, animals, plants, the environment, and by doing so he inspires others to change, to improve consciousness of themselves, and everything that surrounds them. This raises the level of consciousness – it matures the light in us. Let's shine like a lighthouse, because many need our help and guidance, so let's reach out to those who seek and want to move forward.

Life is a game, a beautiful play in which the roles are given, not randomly, but precisely in a way that everybody gets a chance to advance and develop in his/her spiritual path.

There is a divine spark in every man

You can see it in everybody. If you look at things with ease and with love , because deep inside everyone is good, and has a chance to advance and develop.

Man gets wiser, as he ages. Successful homeopathic treatment makes the patient wise and happy. Children, those heavenly beings, full of energy, will and want, can make wonders guided by wisdom of the elderly .Let us be good guides to those little angels.

Be positive, see the beauty. Feel the joy of the sunrise, a bird, a flower, a tree, the sun, the moon, the stars...

Life is full of challenges, and each and every one of

them, makes us learn something , helping us to mature. Embrace them with joy. Where there is peace, there is unity. We are all one.

Illness is a state in which the patient is. The cause itself is very subtle, in the higher levels of our existence, inextensible to our senses.

Only if we get to the very essence of a man, the root of illness can be recognized, and then removed. The root is removed by wisdom, skill and heavenly light.

To get to the essence of man, one should learn watch, and then see. Listen, then hear.

To learn to choose, to connect, to see, to understand, feel, empathies...

During years of our homeopathic practice, we came across a wide variety of human suffering, difficulties, illnesses, disabilities... All of these states limit the man's ability to make, create, develop...

In the course of homeopathic treatment these disturbances of patients' state of health are removed in a swift and easy way. The result often looks like a miracle, but it is in fact a gradual peaceful change, based on the mobilization of the patients own healing powers – immune system.

A change in you changes the world that surrounds you.

if you want a change, change yourself.

Elegant, sophisticated thoughts heighten us.

Learn to be patient, learn to wait...

Create your life yourself. Be courageous.

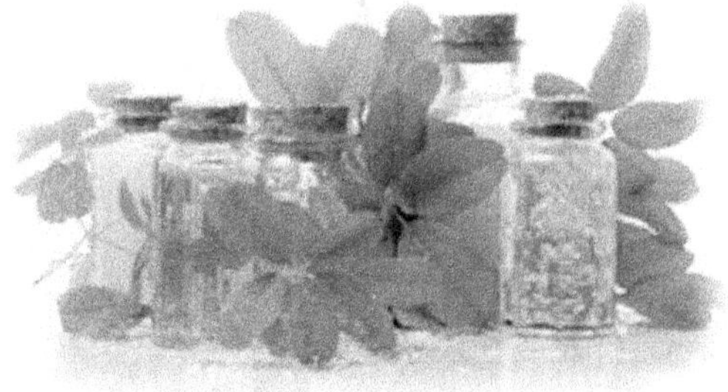

Frequently Asked Questions

Questions of patients about the homeopathic treatment

During the first patients visit in homeopathic treatment – case taking, a series of practical questions are usually asked, about the course of the treatment. These are some of the most frequently asked questions, and our answers:

What does the treatment look like?

The homeopathic therapy starts with case taking.

The patient tells us the reason – discomfort, the illness he comes to treat. He should describe the health issues in his own way, how he feels about them and how they influence him. Besides the finical symptoms it is very important how the patient feels, the way he lives, his mood... The patient should feel free to say what he thinks is important about him, the things that make him different from other people. We talk to him about his prior medical conditions, what he has been through, and, most of all, how did he experience those conditions, and what kind of influence did they have on him. The way he feels about what's happened to him, about his surroundings and, finally, himself, are the most important factors in prescribing the homeopathic therapy.

Who is a suitable patient for homeopathic therapy?

Practically everyone, not just people diagnosed with some medical condition, but anyone who has some kind of disbalance, discomfort, because in this way it is possible to prevent them to develop more serious medical condition. Homeopathic patients are newborns, babies, children, adults, pregnant women, elderly people, animals... A High success rate in homeopathic treatment of the newborns, babies and animals, clearly shows that homeopathic remedy is not based on the placebo effect, because these categories of patients are not even aware they are treated, so any kind of psychological effect on their health status is implausible.

How long does it take to cure a patient with a homeopathic treatment?

The length of treatment depends on the condition of a patient's life force, how long did the condition last, what kind of condition is treated, if the patient is willing to fully cooperate with the homeopathic practitioner...

Which medical condition may be treated with homeopathic medicine?

Homeopathy states that all medical conditions are just a consequence, an expression, of deeper disorders in the patients vital force, so by restoring the vital force to its optimum by a homeopathic treatment any kind of medi-

cal condition may be cured. If the condition of the vital force hasn't deteriorated too much and there is a good cooperation between the patient and homeopathic practitioner, followed by a well suited choice of homeopathic treatment a patient will be cured. Of course, homeopathy is a branch of medicine, so it can't grow a missing limb, but even in cases of physical trauma it may help a lot. Some of the medical conditions treated homeopathically with high success rates are depression, gynecological problems, infertility, asthma, bronchitis, heart diseases, diabetes, autoimmune, allergies, significant improvement in carcinoma...

What may influence the course of homeopathic treatment?

ThThe most important are the factors in the immediate surroundings of the patient, the ones that he is in contact with on a daily bases, such as family members, colleagues at work and work itself, housing conditions, nutrition, lifestyle...

The action of the homeopathic remedy may be diminished by stimulating and toxic substances, in homeopathy referred to as antidotes. A List of these substances should be provided to the patient upon his first visit to a homeopathic practitioner.

Why is it recommended that members of the family also get the homeopathic treatment?

Treatment is more successful if it's range of influence is wider.

The family is an undividable unity of mutual influences. A change, disorder in one family member inevitably causes changes in all. For instance, if a baby is brought to therapy, it is necessary to help the mother first, because the baby is still a part of the mother, especially while very small, so in that period the mothers state is the babies state too, and they are treated with the same homeopathic remedy. It is often enough to give the homeopathic remedy to the mother and the baby gets well without treatment. It is very important how well the pregnancy and delivery went. The Baby is born in a state in which the mother was during the pregnancy. The Mother doesn't often stay in that state after the delivery, because her situation has changed, but the baby may stay in the energy of that state for years, even for a lifetime, limiting its freedom and happiness, and see the world through the prism of that state Homeopathic remedy works on very high levels, and may free a person from the chains of the past. If the whole family is included in the homeopathic treatment, all of them, together get peace, harmony and with it the blessing of health, creation and advancement. The children get healthier, creative, in a higher state of mind.

Why do we schedule follow ups in homeopathic treatment?

In the course of homeopathic treatment the homeopathic practitioner schedules the next follow-up visit, taking into account the state of patients health, his constitution, the type of disorder and, also, the nature of chosen homeopathic remedy. In the meantime, patient may call in for an emergency follow-up.

In the follow-up visit the patient talks about changes in on the mental, emotional and physical level, that he or the people around him have noticed since the last visit. In the beginning they may be very subtle, but paying attention to them is crucial for the further course of the treatment, so the homeopathic practitioner assesses those changes and prescribes the therapy.

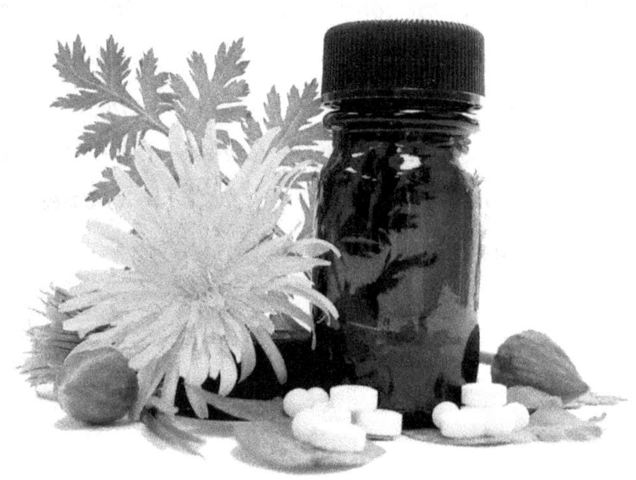

About the Cases

In this book

The cases described in this book illustrate a small portion of successful treatments in years of dedicated team work with Dr. Stojan Primović.

In these cases we have cited the patient's words in case taking and follow ups. It is very important for the homeopathic treatment to pay attention on the exact word that the patient has used, because they show us what the patient really feels, deep inside about himself and his surroundings.

The Patients words in described cases are printed in regular letters, while our thoughts and conclusions are printed in italic.

In this book we have presented twelve cases, where the course of the treatment is given in a condensed form, easier to follow than the original transcripts.

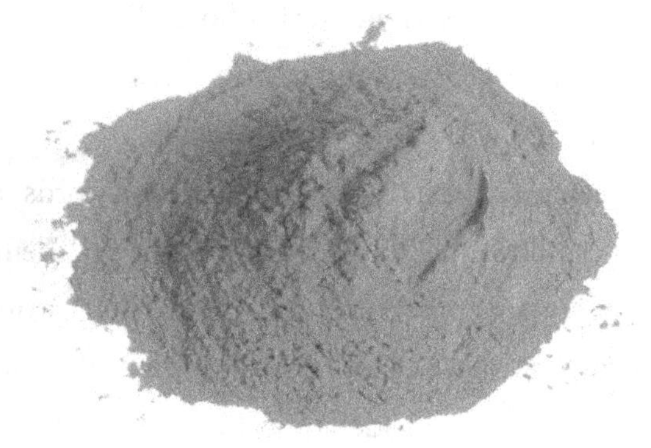

Phosphorus

The Phosphorus Case

A Sixteen year old girl, student

My nose itches, I cough, sneeze... It's some kind of allergy... It starts in November and lasts until February. I also feel like this in August, during the pollination of ambrosia. The allergy first appeared when I was ten, so I have had it for six years, now. I feel itchy in my ears, palate and throat, and my eyes are watery. The secretion looks white and transparent. I have a dry cough during the winter, that keeps me awake all night. When that happened I used Durofilin (generic Theophylline, antiasmathic – bronchospasmolitic). Currently I use Tafen (generic Budesodine, nasal decongestive) when necessary.

I attend a high school in Banja Luka. My average is about 4,5 (B+). In elementary school I had straight A's. Mathematics and physics are the most difficult for me. I would like to study psychology.

When I was seven months old I had a rush that covered my whole body, so I spent seven days in hospital.

I don't like to argue, I'm ok with everybody. I have a boyfriend. He is six years older than me. My parents know about him, but they disapprove. I'm not thinking about marriage. I had my first period three years ago. It is regular, but the first day is painful.

Sometimes I feel my stomach when I get nervous. My feet are often cold.

Since I was seven I have often had headaches, aggravated by the sun and riding on the bus. I often have a headache from the moment I wake up, mostly in the temples, a blunt intensive pain. I may also get a headache if someone wakes me up, all of a sudden.

I am irritable. I can't stand noise and loud music. I feel better when I rap up my head. It goes away when I sleep it off.

I don't like tomatoes. I like warm, salty, spicy food. Milk works well for me, while onions don't. I get a sore throat from soft drinks. I love fish.

Sometimes I get into an argument with my mom, my girlfriend. I just snap, and in a moment I say what I should and shouldn't have, and later I feel sorry for what I said. I get over it fast.

I used to have frequent nosebleeds, on the left nostril.

Rp. Phosphorus C200

Follow-up after one month

My eyes are not itchy and watery anymore and neither are my ears. The next day, after the homeopathic remedy, I got a headache and a sore throat and I could hardly swallow. It turned out to be some kind of flu. I could hardly swallow. It lasted for two days, but even during that period I felt that I had strength, and generally I felt fine. During this last month I had experienced headaches twice, but it didn't last for long, and was less painful than before.

Everything is fine with my boyfriend. We love each

other. My period was a week late this month.

The situation with my mom and dad is also better, even though they are still not very fond of my relationship. I was much more relaxed. I am still very sensitive, but not as much as I used to be.

Day after the administration of homeopathic remedy the patient had a headache that developed in a sore throat, which is a good development, because a chronic condition was transformed into acute, while she was generally fine. Other physical conditions she used to have like itching in nose, eyes and throat had also got better, as well as her psychological condition, so we've decided to,

Rp. Watch and wait

Follow-up after one month

I didn't have hay fever, no itching in the eyes, or ears, and no sneezing. Everything is fine. I didn't have any headaches, even though I ride on a bus to school, for an hour every day… I felt fine…

Rp. Watch and wait

Follow up in six months, or sooner if the patient starts feeling worse physically, mentally or emotionally.

FOLLOW-UP AFTER FOUR MONTHS

I have been fine for the last four months. Lately my nose started to itch. It lasted four five minutes, and then it stopped, and it happened every three to four days...
I had herpes under my nose and on my lower lip, painful when touched.

Before the homeopathic treatment I usually had herpes when I went to the seaside.

Everything else is fine. My period is regular and it's not painful anymore.

Since the itch in the nose has reappeared, and six months has passed since we last administered the remedy, we have decided to repeat the remedy.

Rp. Phosphorus C200

Follow-up after one month

My nose doesn't itch anymore. Everything is great. I'm thinking about my future carrier and studies... Maybe social services... I have tests at school all the time... I only go to school because of my friends... The relationship with my boyfriend is great. We love each other very much.

Since everything is fine, we are going to,

Rp. Watch and wait

Follow-up in six months or when necessary.

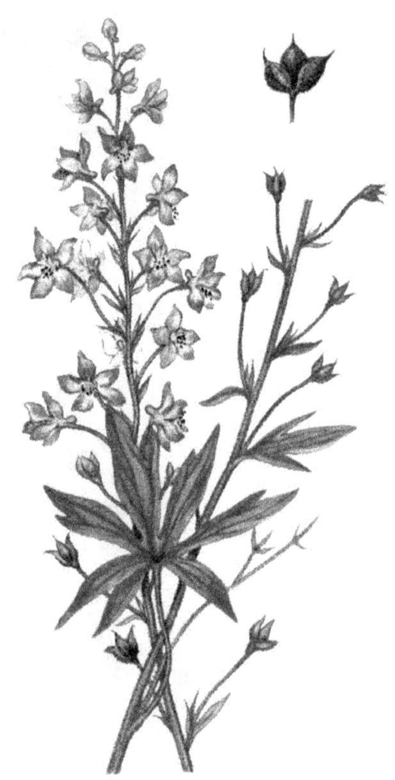

Delphinium staphysagria

The Staphysagria Case

A 34 year old woman, ballet dancer

I came because of a kidney inflammation and Escherichia coli infection in the urinary tract.

Everything started when I caught a cold. I got soaking wet in the rain and caught a draft. It's my fault.

I was taking cold showers after training, walking barefoot...

I had an inflammation of my left kidney, a month and a half ago, with intense pain in the left kidney region and a high fever. I was resting. I felt a pain in my bladder at the end of urination. I was taking antibiotics.

Once I had a sciatica in my back. Now, when I feel pain in my back, I don't know if it's my kidney or sciatica.

I don't feel any intense pains at the moment.

I have a node of fatty tissue on my neck. It hasn't changed in years.

I don't like my job. I was put in charge of finances of a small hotel, and I don't know much about that. I don't like working with numbers. I have three bosses, and each one of them is doing his own thing. You have to twist and turn between their interests. All the workers are suffering because of the situation. I'm trapped with that all day long...

She started crying.

I'm in a dark room. I feel trapped. It suffocates me. Now I am the person responsible for the finances... I used to come to work after eight o'clock in the morning, water the plants, take care of everything as if it were my own home, and everything was fine until I was transferred into the financial section. Now I feel like a puppet, a fool who signs everything, for legitimate and illegitimate businesses.

I have to do everything whatever my managing director orders me to. I get nothing in return. The worst part is that I am the person responsible for the finances! I've lost my identity.

I love making things. Colored photographs, not black

and white! Aesthetics is important to me. In my apartment everything is beautiful. My Photo frames are red, orange… Colors appeal to me.

I dream a lot, in color.

The patient is of delicate stature, oversensitive, she likes beautiful things, flowers, to make, create, she finds colors appealing, she feels trapped at work, forced to do things she doesn't like, and doesn't want to do, but she suffers quietly as all the employees there do... she feels used...

Rp. Carcinosinum desc

Follow-up after one month

I feel great! This is great!

Mentally I feel great. I am much more relaxed!

The first day after the remedy I felt very sleepy.

I almost don't care at all about my job. I don't feel agitated any more. A complete difference! It started right after I took the remedy and it still lasts…

I feel the kidney from time to time, but just in one

spot. Sometimes I feel uneasy at the end of urination.

I dreamt about a herd of white and chestnut horses... It was beautiful.

Considering that the patient's mental state is significantly better, because she is much more relaxed and happier we have concluded that the remedy started the healing process.

Rp. Watch an wait

FOLLOW-UP AFTER ONE MONTH

A month passed. Everything was great. Now my hay fever has started. I used to have it before, but now it's in a much weaker form. I'm in a great mood.

Since the mental state is still good, and she used to have hay fever before, we have concluded that it is a reappearance of old symptoms.

Rp. Watch an wait

Follow-up after one month

Basically I feel fine. I have been anxious lately. My work has started to bother me again and I get anxious for no good reason, but still I see it different than before. It doesn't bother me that much. Outside of work I am fine. Everything is great. I sleep and eat well.

The first remedy was miasmatic, and it worked on deep levels of the past and ancestors, removing the factors that predispose illnesses. Since the mental state is not as good as it was on the last follow up, we have decided to give a remedy of the same miasam, but with a less deep action, a plant with a delicate flower, like she is.

Rp. Staphysagria c200

Follow-up after one month

There is nothing that makes me anxious in my life any more. I don't spend money. Next month I will be relieved of the duty of signing financial documents for my firm, from that responsibility!!!

Something is happening with the node on my neck. It changes in size. It becomes bigger and then smaller.

I have poured out my heart with the things that have bothered me for a while, and since then it has become smaller. I dreamt of horses.

Since everything is going well, she feels better at work, she opened up and became stronger mentally, we have decided to,

Rp. Watch an wait

Follow-up after three months

I have had a boyfriend for six months, now. I feel much better when I am with him. I have some company and support...

I had to go on a business trip for a month. I felt very tense when he was not around. I'm not anxious, but it's hard for me.

I had herpes on my thigh. I used to have it before when I was stressed out or in PMS. Three years ago it was on the front side of my thigh… And it happened to my mother too, at the same time it happened to me!

Since there is a decline in a mental state of the patient, we will repeat the remedy.

Rp. Staphysagria c200

Follow-up after three months

I feel fine. I'm satisfied with myself.

My kidney is fine! Everything is fine!

Only that node of fatty tissue on my neck keeps changing its shape and color. It used to be firmer and bigger, and now it's softer. I feel light tension and burning in that node.

Ten months have passed since the beginning of the therapy... The remedy is good for her. Her mental state is excellent.

Rp. Staphysagria 1M

Follow-up after six months

I feel good, and I am strong both emotionally and mentally. Everything is going according to plan. Everything is fine at work, and the relationship with my boyfriend is great.

Rp. Watch and wait

Follow-up in six months or when necessary.

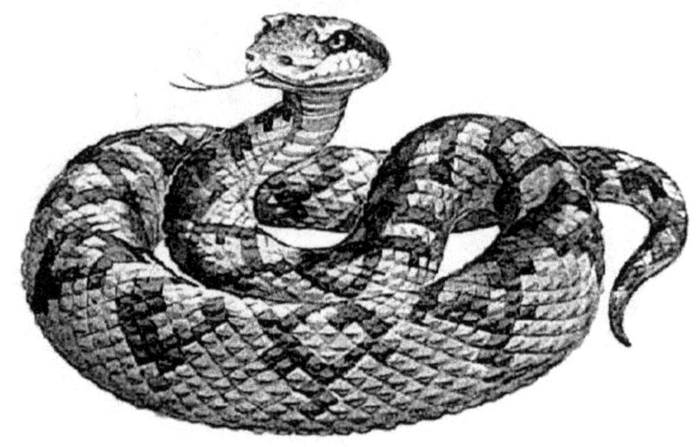

Lachesis Muta

The Lachesis Case

A 60 year old woman, retired

I have had obstructive bronchitis for twelve years. Last year I was in hospital every three months because of my state getting acute. I have a heart condition, too. I was a heavy smoker. I take a lot of drugs: aminofilin (generic aminophylline, antiasmathic), dexason (generic dexamethasone, corticosteroide), berodual inhaler (generic fenoterol, ipratropium, antiasmatic), drugs for my heart condition… I use the inhaler three times in the morning and three times in the afternoon… I had pneumonia, three times fourteen years ago. Before that I had surgery, my appendix was removed. Eight years ago I had a lymphatic node surgically removed from my left armpit. When I was very young I had frequent sore throats. Now I have nodes on my vocal cords.

I live alone. I am retired. I divorced thirty years ago.

I was married for twelve years. I feel scared when I have a choking sensation, I start to shiver, I panic, I have a feeling that it's over, and then I open the balcony. A window must be always opened in my room. I am afraid when I am alone in an elevator and I always wait for someone, so I can go with them.

I feel a spasm in the throat, wheezing, I can't breathe, I have wheezing in my lungs, too. My temperature goes a little above 37°C. I have difficulties to swallowing. When I touch my skin I feel like I'm burning, and I don't have a high temperature. I have some band like formations on my right lung, and circular one on my left lung. On CT x-ray diagnostics it was established that my adrenal glands had stopped working.

Other ways, I was always full of strength. I've never felt cold, and my feet are always uncovered when I sleep. Sometimes I scratch my legs off. I don't wear rings, necklaces or turtleneck sweater, anything that is tight. I always wear shoes on bare foot. Nothing has ever been hard for me to do. I've always liked changes. I used to move furniture around my house. I've traveled a lot. I loved my job, and communicating with people was very important to me. I get agitated by lies, cheating, injustice...

My father had a brain infarction. My mother has tuberculosis of bones; she had her left breast removed because of cancer, cancer of colon and cataract.

Rp. Lachesis C30

Follow-up after ten days

I breathe differently. When I breathe in I feel like my lungs are big. Last four days I didn't take any kind of medications, no pills, nor inhaler... I can't believe it.

In the evening I feel as if I had a temperature in my head and chills in my back. Now I can swallow normally. I can't understand the fact that I can live without inhaler! I walk normally, and I had to stop every once in a while to rest before the remedy...

Rp. Watch and wait

Follow-up after one month

I started to have a productive cough with lots of expectoration. It wakes me up every two to three hours. I feel spasm in my throat, with lots of thick mucus.
I still don't take any medications.

Rp. Lachesis c30

Follow-up after three weeks

I am fine. I feel hot, and sweat a lot, all over my body and around eyes. I feel the need to take off all of my clothes. I wake up at night, because I can't stand the heat. I have energy. I go to bed early, and I wake up around 4 AM. I can breathe fine, and have a productive cough with the expectoration of something white. I feel as if something wants to get out of my throat, like something come out of the right part of my throat, and there is still something on the left.

Rp. Watch and wait

Follow-up after one month

It's high humidity in the air today, and it's hard for me. I can hear myself breathe, with a wheezing sound. I still expectorate thick white mucus.

Everything is fine now on the left side of my throat, but on the right side I feel some kind of node, where the mucus collects, and then I expectorate it out of there… I sweat at night, and get all red in the face.

Apart from that, I have strength, and I am on the move all day long. I don't take any allopathic drugs. Considering the very high humidity in the air today, I feel gre-at.

Before the remedy I would be in hospital due to such weather.

Rp. Lachesis c200

Follow-up after one month

I can breathe better, with less wheezing in my lungs. The mucus I expectorate is less thick, so I can cough it out. The node on the right side of my throat is much smaller. I go somewhere all the time, I'm not at home; I'm on the move. I am a dynamic person, and now I can do all that. When I am at home I like solving crossword puzzles.

Rp. Watch and wait

Follow-up after one month

After the remedy I felt fine.

Yesterday my mom got sick and she was taken to hospital. That stress made my condition worse. It's harder for me to breathe.

I feel like the mucus piles up in the right side of my chest, and suffocates me.

Rp. Lachesis 1M

Follow-up after one week

I breathe better. The node on the right side of my throat is also better, less mucus gathers and I expectorate it. There is no more sweating at night. I am on the move all the time.

Rp. Watch and wait

Follow-up after fifty days

Basically everything is fine. The last two or three days it has been hard for me to expectorate, like the mucus can't move anywhere.

I feel like I have a hoarse voice. I don't sweat. Everything is fine, I just feel as if that mucus is not moving. My breathing is fine, even though the weather is bad for me, there have been weather changes all the time these days.

Rp. Lachesis 1M

Follow-up after two months

I feel great. I have strength. My breathing is good, and I'm active all the time. I've bought a new apartment! I'm very busy moving, and I can manage it…

Now I have strength to help my daughters, if they

need me. I went to visit my daughter in Bosnia. I felt fine during this trip, and before the homeopathic treatment I couldn't make it. Now I live like I used to.

Rp. Watch and wait

Follow-up in three months or earlier if necessary.

The Lachesis Case

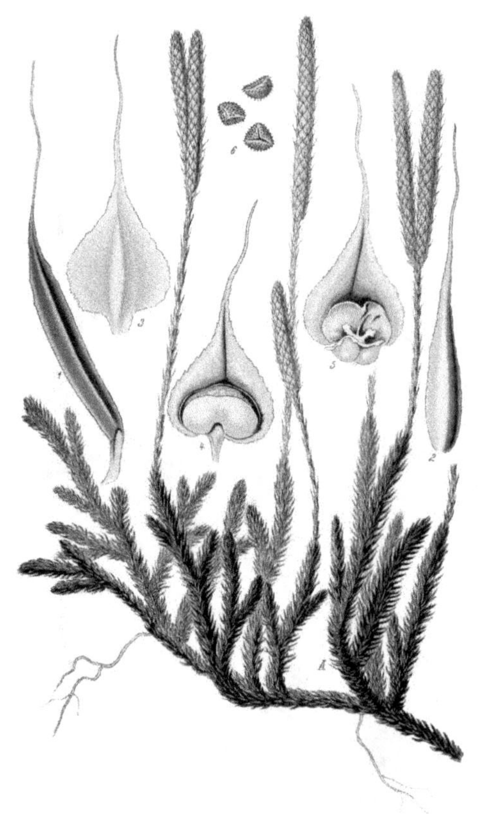

Lycopodium
Clavatum

The Lycopodium Case

A six year old girl

Her mom says:

She has problems with her tonsils. She often has a sore throat, and then she takes antibiotics. She always has a stuffy nose, but with no discharge, so she has some difficulties breathing during the night. She snores and keeps her mouth open. She sleeps with us, and she is restless during her sleep. She doesn't sleep during the day.

She likes to cuddle a lot. She is very shy. She doesn't like boys, because they are naughty, they fight and hit other children. She runs away if she sees a fight. Two or three times she has had nose bleeds. She is in love with a boy, smaller than her! They are the same age…

She goes to ballet. It suits her, because she has the build and talent for dancing. She is fast and slick, compared to other children.

She likes sweets, especially chocolate. She likes strawberries most of all fruits. Her appetite is generally weak. At home her appetite is ok, but in kindergarten she eats almost nothing. I think that's because she is scared of naughty boys there. She is, also, afraid of people especially when they are yelling. Since she has given up a pacifier, she calms down by touching my ears and my husband's.

The girl is very shy, delicately built. She replied very maturely to some of our questions. She is very timid, scared of bigger and stronger people, while she looks down on a boy smaller than she is. She is amative, likes sweets, especially chocolate, has a weak appetite and likes ballet. Based on these observations we recognize an image of a plant with a yellow flower.

Rp. Lycopodium clavatum C30

Follow-up after ten days

She sleeps well, our nights are more peaceful. She breathes well, only her nose is a bit runny. Her tonsils are a bit enlarged, as well as her lymph nodes. She doesn't snore anymore, and doesn't she keep her mouth open.

Her appetite is better, too. She loves cheese, pastry, chicken, fish… She is fast and likes to run. She is more brush, free, courageous than before. We are satisfied.

Since the girl's breathing is better, she sleeps well, she has a good appetite, she is more self-aware and looks bouncy and happy.

Rp. Watch and wait

Follow-up after three weeks

She still breathes well, her appetite is good, she doesn't cry when we take her to the kindergarten, she even eats up everything she gets there for lunch, and it has happened for the first time ever. She mostly eats pastry, just like her dad.

The girl has changed so much for the better, that we could hardly recognize her. She is lively, more communicative than before.

Rp. Watch and wait

Follow-up, when necessary. We have instructed her mother how to recognize when it's time to bring the girl back to us, for repeating the remedy.

Follow-up after six months

Everything had been fine for the last six months. She didn't have a single cold, even though other children her class were ill every once in a while.

Now she has a fever, 38°C. She coughs, sneezes, breathing is more difficult than it was, but not as much as it used to be, but she rather breathes on her nose and mouth at the same time. Her appetite is a bit weaker.

Everything else is fine. She is not in love anymore. She saw the boy she liked, picking his nose and eating it, so she doesn't like him any more...

We find that the immune reaction is very good, because of the high fever.

Generally her state is very good, practically unchanged for the last six months.

Rp. Lycopodium clavatum C200

FOLLOW-UP IN THREE DAYS

The next day after the remedy, she didn't have a fever anymore, and she felt much better. Her nose is not stuffy anymore, so she doesn't have to breathe on her mouth. She coughs less and eats well... She goes to kindergarten.

Everything is fine, and this was just an acute illness, flu. The fact that her immune system cured this flu so quickly, is a sign of a strong vital force...

Rp. Watch and wait

Follow-up, if necessary.

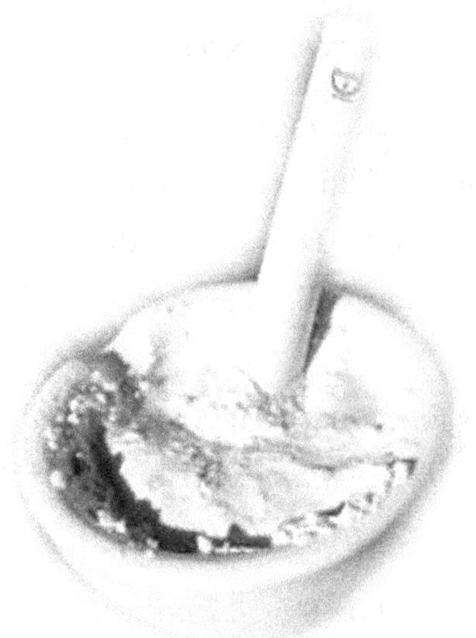

Causticum
Hahnemanni

The Causticum Case

A seventy one year old woman, retired

I came because of a constriction in my throat. The uneasiness moves up from my stomach, and then my throat constricts, so I can't breathe, or talk and everything gets stiff. When I stand up, the vertigo pulls me backwards. When I feel this constriction, I lose my strength. When I get in to this state I scream, and then I can't talk anymore, I lose my ability to speak, as if I was paralyzed. During all that I am always fully aware of everything around me. I always feel like the vertigo pulls me from left to the right. I have been suffering from this for ten years, now. My head is sometimes drawn to one side, with dizziness and stiffne-ss... Sometimes my chin or mouth is drawn to one side. Then I take Bromazepam (generic bromazepam, anxioli-tic), but it doesn't help. In this period I usually have dreams of my loved ones who died. When I get in this state I feel fatigue all the time, and I can't do anything. I just go to my room, to get away from everybody. It forces me to lay down and go to sleep.

It starts with anxiety, then I get tense and restless, I start to shiver and my heart starts pounding. My heart is, other ways, fine, so is my blood pressure. Everything changes in an instant, I get very excited, then I feel this tension and constriction, for 5-10 minutes and then it slowly stops, but I stay restless all day long. My voice starts to shiver. I get fatigue. I avoid people and just sit alone in the room and brood. Then, when the restlessness starts, I walk around the room, doing something, because I can't lie down.

I'm silent by nature. I'm not talkative. I don't reproach, or argue. I rather stay quiet, and then cry it out.

My husband is a little short tempered, so I can't talk back to him, so I just suffer quietly. I get aggravated because my daughter in law takes over my jobs.

My husband's father used to eat my heart out… He was always angry, and liked to insult people, and I am very sensitive to insults. Dishonesty hurts me, and since I am quiet, I can't fight, so I suffer quietly.

My stool is sometimes fine, and sometimes I have diarrhea or I don't have stool for two or three days.

I take Bensedin (generic diazepam, axiolitic) 5-10mg a day.

Based on the patients words, the way she speaks, her dark complexion, the wart on the tip of her nose, the nature of her sensitivity, we recognize an image that fits to the homeopathic remedy:

Rp. Causticum c200

Follow-up after ten days

I feel better! I am satisfied with my life! There has not been a single episode with constrictions and everything that tears me apart!!! No drawing of my chin! These episodes used to make me fatigued, so I had to lie down and sleep, and now I don't have to! Sometimes I wake up at 1 AM, but with no episode. Now I don't have to lie down.

Like something is poking me with a needle and makes me move, so now I work a lot at home all day long... No one can believe it, not even me.

My neighbors in the village can't believe that I am fine and working again. I have more strength and will. I went to visit my neighbors...

I am not taking Bensedin anymore. Now I feel numbness as needles poking me in my legs. Both legs, but more on the left. I feel this numbness in soles, too. I used to feel pain in my left leg before, because I had had surgery on my left hip a long time before...

The patient's state is fantastic. She is in a good mood, has strength, she moves more, sleeps less and she is more social. She doesn't have those episodes that used to threaten her life.

Numbness as needles poking in her legs shows us that the nerves are regenerating and life is getting back in her legs...

Rp. Watch and wait

FOLLOW-UP AFTER THREE WEEKS

I didn't have a single episode. It just starts building up, my heart starts pounding and then it all stops. It happened every three to four days. I have numbness as needles poking me but now just from my knees down, not in whole legs as before.

I have a bit of a back ache. Now, I regularly fall asleep at half past nine, while before I couldn't sleep until midnight.

Her son tells us:

Granny is great! Now she moves around a lot. She is happy. She used to cry a lot in her episodes, when she couldn't speak or do anything. She is active all day long, doing housework, and helping with the calf… Oh, yes, our cow gave birth, so we are all very happy, especially granny.

Since her condition is still very good, and she is in a good mood, she has strength, works, and the symptoms in her legs are moving downwards, we've decided to

Rp. Watch and wait

Follow-up after one month

I still haven't had a single episode. Everything is fine. My legs are still numb, so it makes me difficult to move around. Numbness as needles pinching from my knees down, but they are not cold anymore. I had a bit of a sore throat, like I used to a long time ago, but I didn't have a fever.
My back aches, but not too much.

Since the patient still has difficulties with her legs we have repeated her remedy.

Rp. Causticum c200

Follow-up after two months

No episodes. Right leg is fine, and left one is still a bit numb. Everything else is excellent.

Rp. Watch and wait

Follow-up when necessary.

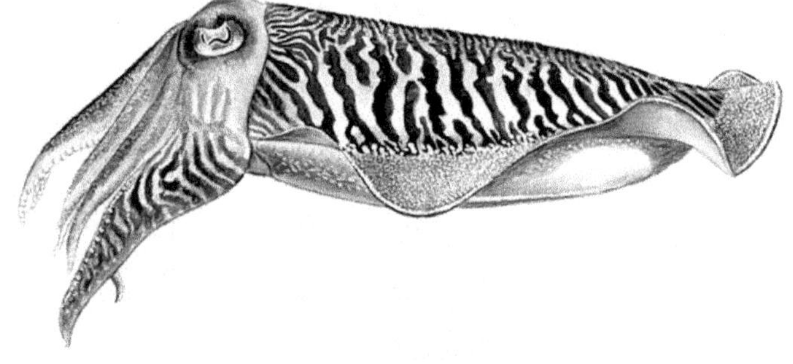

Sepia Officinalis

The Sepia Case

A thirty three year old woman, economist

I have been trying to get pregnant for years, now. I have polycystic ovaries. Escherichia coli was detected on my cervix. I have taken loads of antibiotics up to now, but with no results. I've just got problems with my stomach, too.

I grew up in a village with my mother, who didn't work. As a little girl I used to have a sore throat occasionally, with pustules in my tonsils, so I couldn't swallow. When I was fourteen I had appendicitis.

In high school I was careless, happy and in good health. After I graduated from high school, I went to the Faculty of Social Sciences. I started getting very anxious about my exams… I felt pressure and responsibility.

During my studies I started having dizziness in stressing situations. In that period I was taking Bromazepam for two-three weeks. I also started to have spasms in my cervical muscles. I was going to aerobic classes four times a week… That helped me to feel quite well again.

Then I got married.

After the wedding I was getting stressed out about finding an apartment, and that I should have children… I stopped going to aerobic, because I just couldn't find time. Then the dizziness and neck pain started again. In all that mess I'm not getting pregnant and the pressure on me is rising.

At work I'm in an office all day long and I feel that closed spaces suffocate me. Then, six months ago I lost my brother, as doctors said, after the routine operation of a cyst in the pancreas… That finished me off.

After that I started having stomach pains. My husband and I have helicobacter pylori and we have taken a huge amount of antibiotics, but I still suffer the same pains. I don't want to drink those drugs anymore. I feel pressure in my intestines when I bend forward.

Then I caught a cold. My legs were frozen, so I saw

blood when I urinated and I felt pain during urination, especially at the end of urination. I have a period about every 50-60 days. I am chilly. My legs are always cold, as well as my hands. My parents' health is quite all right. My mom has Cervical Spondylosis, and my dad has had thrombosis since he was 25, but they function just fine…

Since the patient is chilly with cold feet and hands, and she feels better from vigorous physical activity, she has polycystic ovaries, feeling of pressure, physically strong, having late periods, as well as the way she behaved in first contact with us, where she was unpleasant, suspicious, angry, very inaccessible, so we have decide to give her the homeopathic remedy,

Rp. Sepia officinalis C200

Which turned out to be true and you will see why

Follow-up after one month

The remedy suited me great. I was very sleepy. The first day after the remedy I had a little headache. The relationship with my husband was excellent. We went for a walk in the countryside. I love to take walks and it suits me very well.

My hands and feet are warm now!

I got my period on 38th day. About the middle of my period I got some mucous reddish secretion, and in PMS my breasts didn't hurt.

Everything is going good, so we have decided to give a higher potency of the remedy.

Rp. Sepia officinalis 1M

Follow-up after one month

Now my period lasts for 30 days. I went to the ultrasound, and on the 10th day a follicle was detected. Before the remedy I hadn't had follicles. We were making a baby! Echerichia coli was found in my urine, but I don't have any symptoms. My mood is great! It can't be better.

Since she feels good emotionally, she has a follicle, she generally feels good, and the presence of Escherichia coli we see as a cleansing of the urinary system, we have decided to,

Rp. Watch and wait

FOLLOW-UP AFTER ONE MONTH

I am pregnant!!! I've had some reddish secretion on 21st day of my cycle, and I felt as if I was going to get my period, it scared me a bit, but it turned out to be a false alarm.

I feel a little nauseous. I mostly eat salty and sweet. We are so happy now!

Since everything is excellent,

Rp. Watch and wait

FOLLOW-UP AFTER ONE MONTH

I am two months pregnant now. All the test results were fine, except for the thyroid gland where TSH (thyreostimulating hormone) was a little higher. I was at mom's and dad's, everything reminded me of my brother, and that shook me up. I've had bad dreams. I have fears if everything is going to be ok with my pregnancy, and if I will have to take some medication. I have nausea and sometimes I throw up, usually in the evening. I'm oversensitive to smells. My digestion is a bit weak. I feel some kind of panic when I have to go to the doctor's.

Since the patient's mood and emotional state is worse, she is stressed out about her brother's death again and she is afraid of doctors, we have decided to repeat the remedy.

Rp. Sepia officinalis 1M

We've advised the patient about the healthy diet that fits her constitution, her current state, season, choice of food and way of preparing the food...

Follow-up after one month

I am three months pregnant now. I still work a little on some things, and then I plan to go to my parents in the countryside. Car exhaust gases suffocate me. I have mild nausea. I feel stabile. All of my test results are good. I'm planning a natural birth.

Everything is going as planned...

Rp. Watch and wait

Follow-up after one month

I am four months pregnant now. I don't have nausea anymore. Smells still bother me. My hands and feet are warm. The test results for the thyroid gland are outstanding. I'm fine.

Everything is good, so

Rp. Watch and wait

Follow-up after three months

I am seven months pregnant now. I was in the countryside twice for two weeks each time. The baby has 1.4 kg. We had the anniversary of my brother's death... I took it well. My gums bleed a little. I still follow your instructions about diet and lifestyle. Generally, I feel fine.

Everything is on track, so

Rp. Watch and wait

Follow-up after one month

I am eight months pregnant now. Nothing bothers me now, so I am finally enjoying my pregnancy. I walk a lot, 4 to 5 km a day. I don't have swellings. I feel a little back pain. We're slowly getting ready… My husband is ok.

Rp. Watch and wait

Follow-up after one month

I am nine months pregnant now… Everything is fine… I'm in a good mood. We can't wait to see the baby! I've decided to have a natural birth.

Since there are no hospitals in Serbia where a homeopathic practitioner could assist his patient during birth, we have prepared for her a set of homeopathic remedies, with detailed instructions how and when to take these remedies before, during and after delivery. We have also instructed her, what to do in certain possible states after giving birth...

Follow-up – Baby

Mom came to show us her baby.

We came with the baby to meet our doctors! She was born on February 10th, so she is Aquarius like you! A child of the future. She is now a month and a half old.

She doesn't sleep much, and she cries when she wakes up. She has stomach cramps at the beginning of breastfeeding.

She hasn't had any rashes until now. Her face is red. We think that this eczema is from peanuts, because I ate a lot of it...

When she nurses her head becomes a bit wet at the nape. Her stool is fine, twice a day, yellow, a bit soft. She's been given two vaccine shots up to now.

Rp. Calcarea carbonica C30

We have given some advice to the mother's diet during breastfeeding, what kind of balm to use for wiping the baby's bottom, what herbal teas to give to the baby.

We also instructed the mother how to recognize the baby's states in which she should come to us.

FOLLOW-UP – BABY AFTER THREE DAYS

The baby is just fine. Her face is nice and clean. Two or three hours after the remedy eczema started to redraw. Cramps are better, too.

Rp. Watch and wait

FOLLOW-UP – BABY AFTER FOUR MONTHS

Baby is seven months old now. She is mostly fine. She sweats a lot and often cries breathless!

She wants to be gently rocked in my arms. She has become short tempered, and her every wish has to be fulfilled.

She likes to eat, she is impatient and ravenous. Her palms

and soles get all wet when she's nursing.

Rp. Chamomilla c30

FOLLOW-UP AFTER ONE WEEK

She doesn't cry breathless anymore. She has matured, and now she uses the potty. She started teething when she was six months old, and for now, she's got two teeth. She had a bit of an increase in salivation, but now she's fine. Everyt-hing else is fine, too. She is in a good mood. She likes other children...

Rp. Watch and wait

FOLLOW-UP – MOTHER

A year after delivery, I am still breastfeeding my baby. I felt great until now. My feet are getting a bit colder... I have some secretion in my vagina... I got my period six months after delivery. It's not very regular... Other ways I am fine.

Rp. Sepia officinalis 1M

Follow-up after three months

Both me and my baby are fine. We are one whole. Together with daddy we are a happy family…

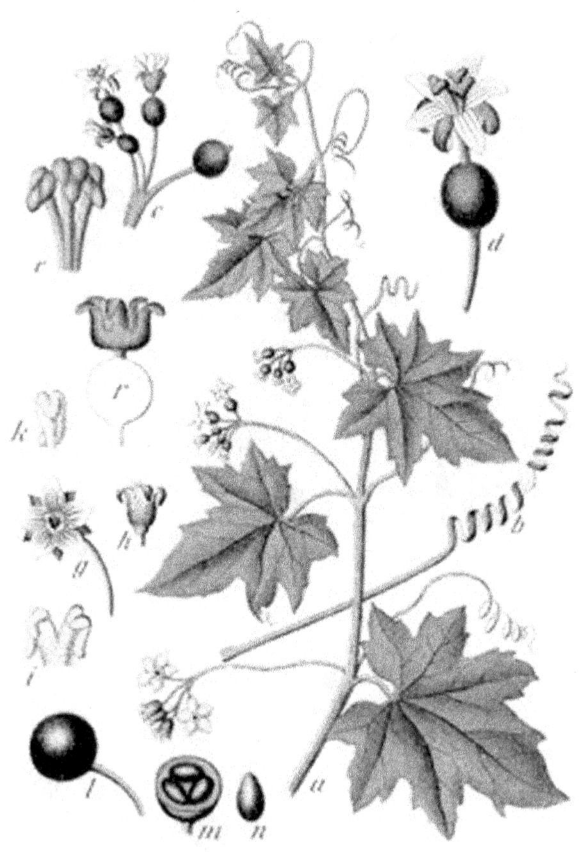

Bryonia Alba

The Bryonia Case

A twenty five year old man, athlete

I have had frequent and severe migraines for seven years now. It started nine years ago. These migraines always start in the morning, as soon as I open my eyes, no matter what time it is. Sometimes it starts at once, and sometimes gradually. When it starts I just don't know where I am. I vomit and I can't talk. I feel heaviness in my eyelids. I have to lie down in a dark, quiet room, without distractions. I can't move. I had my last migraine attack a few days ago. I took pain killers but they didn't help me much. A neck massage helps me reduce the pain. My mother has had migraines all her life.

I am a sportsman and I had some injuries. My left shoulder was operated twice, because of a ruptured muscle that made my shoulder dislocate easily. Now my arm is fine.

Then I was injured when I went skiing. I hit my back on a rock, and I just lied there. It was a blunt trauma to lower back. I couldn't feel my legs.

I am warm blooded. It does me good to drink a glass of cold water in large draughts.

I usually drink a lot of water. I like sweets, cakes and chocolate. I am short tempered, but I keep it under control.

I get angry in a second, and it ends up in a conflict, aggression, and it's a shame because I am basically very protective. When it starts I get anxious, biting, the pressure in my head is as if it will burst.

The presence of headache that gets worse from moving, noise, and being ameliorated by peace, drinking cold water, a person who appears to be calm in compensated state, being warm blooded, all together best fits to the picture of homeopathic remedy English mandragore, so

Rp. Bryonia alba c30

Follow-up after ten days

I came home and soon after I fell asleep. It was about half an hour after taking the remedy. I felt more relaxed and calmer.

The second and third day everything was fine, and then the fourth day in the morning the headaches started, but it didn't last as long as it used to and I didn't vomit. The symptoms were much milder.

Next day everything was fine, but the following morning I got a headache again, but also much milder than I used to have before.

And so it went on, practically every other day. I used to have a severe headache once a month, and now they are more frequent, but with far milder symptoms.

The remedy has started the process of healing. There are evident changes in his physiology. We will repeat the remedy but in a higher potency.

Rp. Bryonia alba C200

Follow-up after seven days

At first I felt great. I was working a lot and I was very active. I didn't have a headache for a few days.

Everything was fine and then this morning the pain was back as it used to be before the first remedy. I was so nauseous that I almost vomited. I could hardly get here. I can't stand any kind of movement; everything is the same as it was before...

The patient is in aggravation, and since his current state is hard to bear, we are giving him the same remedy in high potency.

Rp. Bryonia alba 10M

And we've got immediate amelioration.

Follow-up after two months

Soon after I got the remedy I fell asleep. I woke up as good as new.

Since then I haven't had a headache, and now two months have passed! I feel good. Business is also going well for me.

I'm going to get married in a month. I feel great!

The remedy has successfully worked on high levels. The patient is not only better physically, but also mentally and emotionally. Since the patient had several sports injuries in the past, we are considering giving him a remedy for those conditions, but for now, since he feels fine we

Rp. Watch and wait

FOLLOW-UP AFTER THREE MONTHS

Three months have passed. I got married. Business is going well. I don't have headaches anymore. Sometimes I feel pain in my operated shoulder when the weather changes.

Now it's the right time to give him a remedy for unhealed traumas from the past. We are giving him

Rp. Arnica montana 10M

Follow-up after one month

For the first few days after the remedy I dreamt of some things from the past, exactly from the period when I was training. After that I felt pain in my left shoulder for one whole day, and then it stopped. After that the backache started, exactly in the same place I hit my back on the rock, for half a day. Now everything is fine.

The remedy has cured the old wounds, in order stated in Herrings "laws" from top to bottom, and in the reverse order of their appearance upon the body.

We are satisfied with the state of our patient and we have told him to call for Follow-up if he feels any kind of difficulties – physical, mental or emotional. He should come for Follow-up, anyway, in six months or a year, so that we see if it's necessary to repeat his remedy, if there are changes on subtle levels that can only be detected by an educated homeopathic practitioner, because it's best to give the remedy on time.

With regular Follow-ups and repeating constitutional

remedy at the right moment, the patient gets a chance to keep his state of well-being, peace, balance, efficiency in business and everything else he wishes.

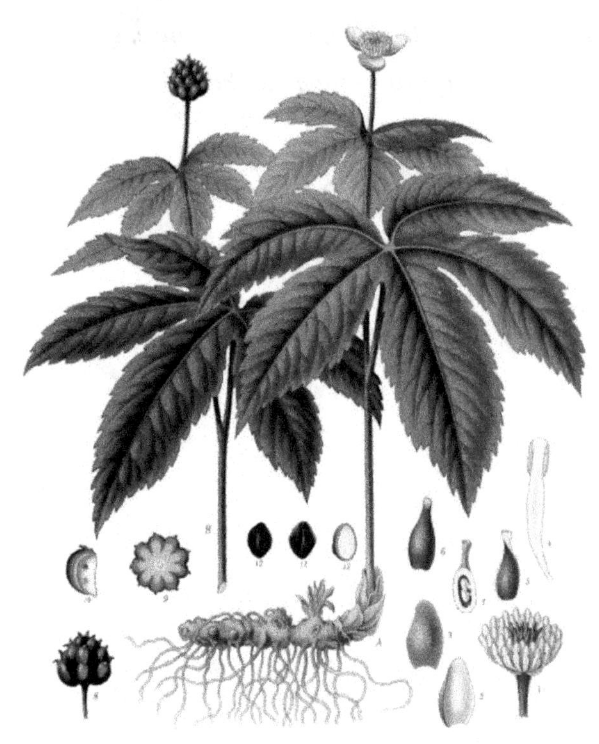

Hydrastis
Canadensis

The Hydrastis Case

A thirty six year old woman, accountant

I am an accountant in a firm, and I work all day long. I live with my fourteen year old daughter, mom, dad and sister.

This drug makes me tired all the time, but without it I can't get out of the house, not even to the grocery's.

I can't do ordinary things, like I can't take the bus, can't stand in a queue, when I see people, commotion, something happens as if my blood pressure goes down, my mind goes blank for a moment, I start to sweat and take my clothes off. My heart rate increases, with fear of something, someone.

I fainted for the first time when I was nineteen.

It all started five years ago when some people around me were arrested. I keep imagining a possible confrontation with the law. It haunts me.

It happened for the first time when I was driving my car. I had to stop and get out.

I felt some kind of pain throughout my body, in my heart, like some kind of heat. I went to a psychiatrist, and he gave me Prozac (fluoksentin, antidepressive) and I was taking it for a month and after that Rivotril for four years now.

I can't stand the sun, I avoid it. I drink a lot of water, I'm always thirsty. My upper lip moves involuntarily.

I want to stop using Rivotril and get well.

The combination of constitutional and iatrogenic conditions in our patient is a result of taking Rivotril, so we have decided to start the treatment by treating this secondary condition, and only after that we can expect to get the picture of her underlying condition.

Based on her posture, like she is ready to jump at any moment, by the modality that she feels worse from heat, agoraphobia, panic attacks, we have decided to start with homeopathic remedy arg-nit.

Rp. Argentum nitricum c200

Follow-up after four days

After the remedy I had a terrible headache, so for the first time I didn't go to work.

The next day I went to work, but my manager was yelling at me, so I went home early. I was bothered by people and noise, on a bus. I couldn't eat, so I took Rivotril.

Since the patient had a substantial reaction to the remedy, a headache on the first day, we will repeat the remedy in a higher potency.

Rp.Argentum nit 1M

Follow-up after ten days

I'm on sick leave. I haven't taken Rivotril for five days. My old symptoms have returned today, the same symptoms that made me go to a psychiatrist at that time. I work, but it's like I have late reactions, a confusion in my head. I have to sit down, bend my head forwards and close my eyes. I have to believe that my space is not in danger and that no one's watching, because it would bother me, like some kind of fear. It's as a semiconscious state, like someone is holding my occiput. My calf muscles on both legs are cramped, as is the tip of my tongue. I feel as if I'm not in coordination with myself. My sensitivity to smell has increased. My skin is dryer, tensed, like it's about to crack.

When I move my head, I feel like my brain is spinning. My hands are shivering and I feel fatigued and sweaty. Now I couldn't go out even if I had to.

My boss doesn't have any understanding.

At home, I do all the work. My sister doesn't mind the mess…

Everything is going exactly as we expected! The layer of disturbance caused by Rivotril is removed and we can now see the picture of the underlying disease. Based on her old fashioned look, tidiness', hardworking nature, long hair pined in a classical manner, some kind of rightful harshness and decisiveness we have decided to give her the homeopathic remedy,

Rp. Hydrastis canadensis c200

Follow-up after ten days

I'm not taking Rivotril anymore! The very first day after the remedy I was already feeling fine. After three days I was perfectly well, as if a burden had been lifted off my chest. I feel as if I can do anything! I received a job offer, in another city. I will stay there for five days, and I'll go home on weekends. My daughter can stay with her grandfather and grandmother. She is fifteen years old! I will do my job in better conditions, for a better salary.

I'm thinking about saving money for a car. I haven't driven a car for four years... I get up with ease. I sleep well. A significant difference!!!

Since she is fine we,

Rp. Watch and wait

Follow-up after three weeks

Everything is great. I feel fine. I'm going to start my new job next month. I feel significantly better, I can work and achieve more. In the morning I get up with ease.

I feel stable, but I still can't get used to it. My period used to be more frequent, and now it's normal. I feel fantastic, as I used to be.

Rp. Watch and wait

Follow-up after two months

Everything is still great. I'm in a good mood. My life is back on track. I feel great about my new job, too.

Rp. Watch and wait

Follow-up in three months or sooner if necessary

Follow-up after three months

I feel fine. I feel absolutely stable. I feel as if I were born again, nothing is too hard for me now, everything is easy, no anxiety…

I feel great. My boss has doubled my salary, just to keep me on my job, so I've decided to stay.

Rp. Watch and wait

Follow-up when necessary.

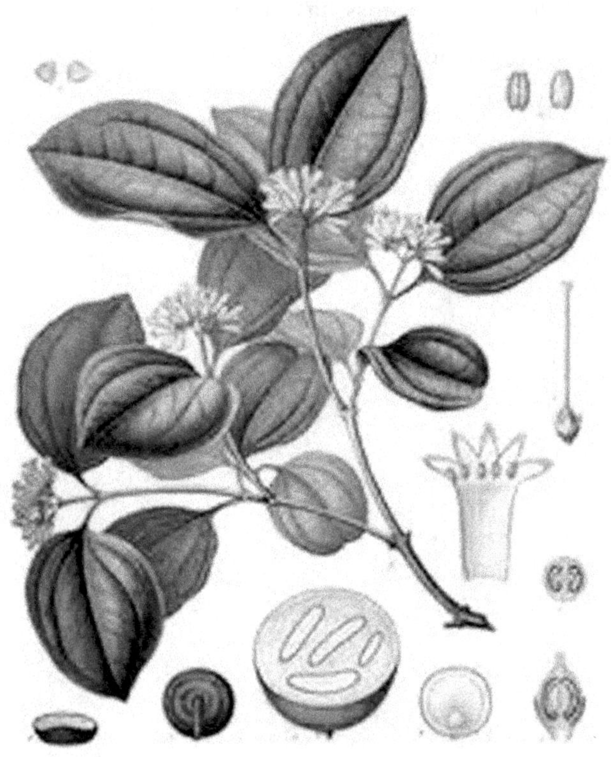

Nux Vomica

The Nux Vomica Case

A sixteen year old boy, student

I came because of my acne. They appeared in my junior year, a year ago. The acnes first appeared on my forehead, then on my chin and on my cheeks. Acnes get bright red, and after they heal, pigmentation spots are left in their place. I went to a beautician, took antibiotics, mostly Dovicin (generic doxycycline, antibiotic), but nothing helped.

My mom told me that my birth went well, but when I was four months old I barely stayed alive, because I got Haemophilus influenzae and a severe pneumonia, so I was treated with a pile of penicillin, and after that my asthma started and all those exhausting inhalations. That's how I spent the first three years of my life. I didn't go to kindergarten, so I didn't get any of children's diseases, not even chicken pox.

Now I'm training basketball. It's very important to

me. It's great. I would like to become a professional in some good basketball club. I'm 190cm tall. I'm good at it, can't say the same thing about school. I got an F in two classes lately. I know I should raise my grades, but I just can't. I get a terrible anxiety in those classes. I argue with my parents twenty times a day. I have stage fright, my palms get sweaty and I shiver like I'm cold.

I don't feel comfortable in front of the girls because of my acne. I don't like the people in my new school. There is a bunch of bullies, who molest everybody, and also the gossiping... All of that bothers me. School is very stressful for me.

I like to eat sweets, chocolate and crepes with chocolate most of all. I also like pizza and all kinds of meat.

His mother says:

It's chaos at home. I argue with my son all the time. Sometimes he gets so agitated that he starts throwing things, anything he can get a hold of. Horrible! Those acnes have a very bad influence on him. One day a lot of acnes appeared on his face, he didn't even go to school, because he didn't want the girls to see him like that. He spent the whole afternoon sitting on a wall all alone, instead of going to school. He has a troublesome friend whom he protects all the time. We argue about that, too... We are afraid that he might end up with people who might have a bad influence on him... Please try to have an influence on him so he can come to his senses.

We have realized that this boy is a very sensitive person, that he cares a lot about his friends, their opinion of him, that he has abrupt reactions and fits of anger, a reflection of the fact that he is powerless to change the situation that doesn't suit him.

He is in some kind of teenage rebellion. He is very fast and skillful, and that makes him so successful in sports. His skin eruptions are in a way very much alike the anger that pours out of him. When we talk to him, we feel his inner anxiety and impatience.

Rp. Nux Vomica C30

We also gave an explanation to his mother that home-

opathic treatment should start healing process as well as opening ones consciousness, by giving a homeopathic remedy.

Follow-up after three weeks

My face is less flashed. I'm in conflict with my dad. I said a lot of things I shouldn't have. My friends bother him, and it makes me very frustrated. My friend lives with his mom and granny. My dad thinks that he's a hooligan…

His dad has joined the therapy, and he adds:

He is more responsible, but his behavior is still horrible. He behaves like a bully, he's even worse, with fits of anger, he threatens that he will leave home, he insults, swears, his mother cries…

The remedy has started the healing process, opened the case, everything that was suppressed has surfaced and everybody has started talking sincerely...

Rp. Nux Vomica C200

Follow-up after three weeks

My face is better, the discoloration spots are peeling off and there is no new acne coming out… I am happier, and it's easier for me to see other people… Everything is ok with girls. I've managed to pull up my grades. The atmosphere in classes is better... I don't argue that much with my mom and dad anymore. There are misunderstandings here and there, but far less than before. My appetite is better. Everything is great at basketball training!

Rp. Watch and wait

Follow-up after two months

My face is much better. I look less flashed and I don't have the kind of acne I used to. There is an acne here and there, but it heals pretty fast, but before my whole face would be covered with acne. The atmosphere at home is ok. We all get along much better. I still have an F in two classes, and that bothers me…

We have decided to raise the potency of the remedy. We expect even better emotional state.

Rp. Nux Vomica 1M

Follow-up after two months

I was at the seaside. It was very nice. My face is great! I have a girlfriend. I have more self-esteem. I've found some new friends. Everything is great.

Rp.Watch and wait

Follow-up after one month

I have a sore throat and it aches when I swallow, as if I had a lump in my throat. It aches even when I yawn. It started three days ago. At first I felt some kind of rawness in my throat. Now the ache in my throat wakes me up at night and my mouth gets dry...

I feel better during the day. Pustules have appeared on my tonsils. I felt this way two years ago, and then I took antibiotics.

Generally I feel great, I have energy and I'm in a good mood. Oh, yeah! I've almost forgotten to tell you that I got some rash on my back, just like the one I had had four years ago.

I've managed to pull up my grades in those two classes where I had F's.

Some old suppressed diseases surfaced, so we decide to,

Rp. Watch and wait

Follow-up after six months

I feel fine. My face is great. I go to school. Everything is fine with my friends and everything else has somehow got better, too. At home everything is fine as well, we get along much better, we talk more, there is much more love. I'm satisfied.

Rp. Watch and wait

Follow-up in six months, or sooner if necessary.

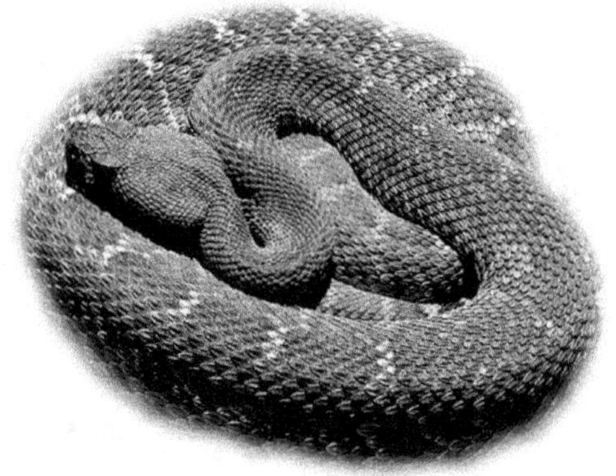

Crotalus Cascavella

The Crotalus Cascavella Case

A fifty five year old woman, secretary

I have had this problem for more than ten years. I've tried many things, but nothing helped. I feel a terrible burning pain in my mouth. I feel like my mouth is full of stinging nettles, so I feel burning under my tongue, palate and throat around the tonsils. I can't eat anything. I have a node in my throat that sometimes shows up and is visible. I sometimes get a lockjaw, so I can't open my mouth. At that time my salivary glands get swollen and any kind of taste irritates me, even mild ones. I was on a liquids only diet. My mouth gets dry even though I drink enough water.

I am a loner. I don't like to go out. I get a high blood pressure every time I have to go somewhere. I don't like crowds. I get scared easily, so I get excited and my heart starts pounding faster… Sometimes I start laughing like a child, and other times I get silent and I just can't say a word. I became undisciplined. I used to fight for the things I cared about, and now nothing.

My eyes are protruded. I didn't have that before menopause. I've had a laryngeal nerve inflammation and trigeminal neuralgia. I have vocal cord nodules. Now I feel the pain mostly in my jaw joint and it starts in the morning when I wake up, followed by a shiver and increased heart rate.

I don't get my period anymore. Sometimes I get heat flushes. For two or three days I have about five heat flushes during the day, and, let's say three more at night, followed by a few days without any heat flushes.

I often have a high blood pressure, up to 215 over 120 mmHg. I also had arrhythmias at that time. I wake up with my heart pounding like an animal's.

I was taking lots of allopathic remedies, poisoning myself, like different kinds of antidepressants, mostly Rivotril (Clomazepam, antiepileptic). I'm not taking it at the moment. Right now I'm taking Presolol (Metroprolol, beta-adrenergic blocker), Prilazid (Cilazapril, antihypertensive) and Demetrin (Prazepam, anxiolytic).

The patient gave us the impression of an anxious, impulsive person of high energy, with swift reactions. Considering the presence of fear and restlessness in our patient, we have decided to start the treatment with a remedy for acute states:

Rp. Aconitum napelus 1M

FOLLOW-UP AFTER TEN DAYS

I feel a bit better. I have some hope after a long time. I am calmer and less anxious.

I still feel the pain, but it's not as intensive as it used to be. As soon as I wake up and my salivary glands start to work, I begin to feel the pain in the jaw joint and I can't talk. I have to be careful when yawning, because my jaw joint used to dislocate before. I feel a strong physical pain. I suffer a lot. The pain is stronger on the left side and it gets worse when I move. That pain from the jaw joint irradiates deep in to my ear. I lie down like a plank with my eyes closed, like in a plaster cast. As the pain intensifies, I start losing my strength, so I have to lie down like that, I start shivering and I get icy cold, especially my face. I fast in those days and I can't eat anything. When I'm not in pain, I eat five times a day. I'm afraid of getting a stroke, of being disabled…When I bend down to tie my shoe laces, the blood rushes in to my head. I feel worse on rainy days.

I sometimes feel a pain shooting across my heart and stomach. I feel as if I have a hole in my stomach and I don't have any energy.

My parents have literally poisoned me with stories about death, and how they don't want to live anymore.

I can't stand aggression and rudeness. It eats me up when I see such a behavior.

When I walk bare foot on small pebbles I get dark red bruises and spots. I feel worn out and molested. I feel as if I was always just giving, without getting anything in return. All of my health issues started with menopause. Until then I was ridiculously healthy.

Based on her appearance, the way she talks, the presence

of some kind of aggression and the words with which she described her state, the intensity of symptoms we have decided to give her a remedy from the animal kingdom which suits her best.

Rp. Crotalus cascavella c30

Follow-up after three days

I feel very good!

The very first evening after the remedy the pain decreased to minimum. Next morning I woke up with the pain, and then I went back to bed and the pain passed! That had never happened before. I was up all day, working...

A dark spot appeared on my right leg and that is something that had happen to me before. I also got acne in two places on my leg and that happened before.

Today, the third day after the remedy it happened! My salivary glands were not swollen after such a long time! I was crying with joy!

My blood pressure is still high, about 180 over 105

mmHg, but it's much better than before. My heart is pounding and I feel a pressure like a ball in my head, with shivering.

My life is much better without that pain.

After a short aggravation came amelioration and some old symptoms have returned. Her mood is much better, so

Rp. Watch and wait

FOLLOW-UP AFTER TEN DAYS

This is worth living for!!!

First day after Follow-up everything was great. In the evening I just felt some pressure in the right jaw joint, but insignificant. I lied down and fell asleep. In the morning my salivary glands were just a little swollen, with some pain here and there, and then it went away.

I don't have heat flushes. No pulsating in my head, either. My heart doesn't pound like it used to, and I didn't feel high blood pressure.

For the last two days I've had cramps in my right leg when I lie down. I used to have that to a long time ago.

We took her blood pressure after the Follow-up and it was 160 over 90 mmHg. Since her mental and emotional state is fine, the pain is far less intense and rare with return of old symptoms, we've decided to,

Rp. Watch and wait

Follow-up after two weeks

I have been feeling fine for the last ten days, like I have never felt before!
Mentally and emotionally I feel great. I slept well. I have been waking up every morning with no pain or heart pounding.
My husband said:
"You were walking on the edge and these people have brought you back to life. You are a completely different person now. You are like you've use to be."

I had been perfectly fine until yesterday morning, when I felt a little pain that lasted for a while, and then it faded away. It was the same this morning...

We've decided to raise the potency of the remedy.

Rp. Crotalus cascavella c200

Follow-up after three weeks

My first reaction on the remedy was great!

The mild pain that was coming back for a few days before the Follow-up, has completely gone!

I was fine until a few days ago when the old pain in my vocal cords came back. I feel as if they were on fire. I feel the pain deep inside my ear and throat. I used to have that too.

My salivary glands are a bit swollen, but far less than before.

I've felt intense burning from the inside. It burns so hard like the bile. Last few days my legs have been restless in bed. I have cramps in my muscles. That happened for the first time two or three years ago.

It feels like someone is biting you. Everything was eating me up and drained me. I'm not dying, and on the other hand I feel like my life is stuck up my ass...

The patient has completely opened to us. She started expressing herself freely and talking sincerely. Since the treatment is on a good course, and those old unhealed illnesses are coming back to surface, and that she is emotionally a bit unstable, anxious and excited, we have decided to raise the potency of the remedy.

Rp. Crotalus cascavella 1M

Kontrola nakon tri nedelje

I feel truly superb mentally and emotionally. I'm great now. I used to be depressed, drinking lots of alcohol, poisoning myself for years. Now I don't drink. I'm not nervous, nor depressed.

I feel a pain in my throat like I felt at the time when I had my tonsils removed. When I start talking I have a mild hoarseness, but after a few words it fades away. The acne on my leg has reappeared.

Since the mental and emotional state is great, and old suppressed illnesses are coming back to surface and healing, we've decided to,

Rp. Watch and wait

Follow-up after one month

I was at the seaside for ten days. I felt great every single day!

I felt a bit worse on the fifth day, in the middle of vacation, but I got well very fast, so I felt great again!

I didn't get sun allergy, and I had had it for 20 years! I'm truly amazed!

I had a cramp in my calf a few times when I starched my leg. I felt like everything went downwards into my legs… I walked bare foot on small pebbles on the beach, but I didn't I get any bruises.

My heart is fine as well as my blood pressure. I feel so much better than before.

Since the patient is fine,

Rp. Watch and wait

Follow-up after two months

I feel fine. I'm in a good mood. I'm free from pain.

It has been raining a lot lately, yet I feel fine. Before the homeopathic treatment I would have suffered like a maggot in such a weather.

I sometimes get a dark acne on my leg.

My heart is fine, as well as my blood pressure.

Since the patient's state is really well, eruptions are appearing on her skin and everything is going according to the Herring's law, so we have decided to

Rp. Watch and wait

Follow-up after three months

For the first two months everything was great, even though I had lots of work and action in that period. Last month some old issues at home came to the surface, so I was a bit upset. For a few nights I had trouble sleeping, and in the morning my heart started pounding, but not as hard as it used to. My salivary glands got swollen a little and the pain reappeared. It was mild and it disappeared quickly, in half an hour... It wasn't exactly a pain but more like unease, but it's all great compared to what it used to be.

Since the patients mental and emotional state has declined a bit, we have decided to repeat the remedy in the same potency as the last time.

Rp. Crotalus cascavela 1M

Follow-up in six month, or earlier if necessary

FOLLOW-UP AFTER SIX MONTHS

I felt great. My life's got meaning once again. I started doing things that I had neglected for a long time because of my condition. I enjoy all that. My daughter gave birth. I was able to help her a lot and that makes me very happy. I've made through all of that excitement and action about the baby… I've had strength and energy… All together I've had a nice time.

Everything is really good, so we,

Rp. Watch and wait

We have also instructed the patient on which symptoms she should pay attention in order to come to Follow-up in an optimal time to get the remedy, when and if necessary.

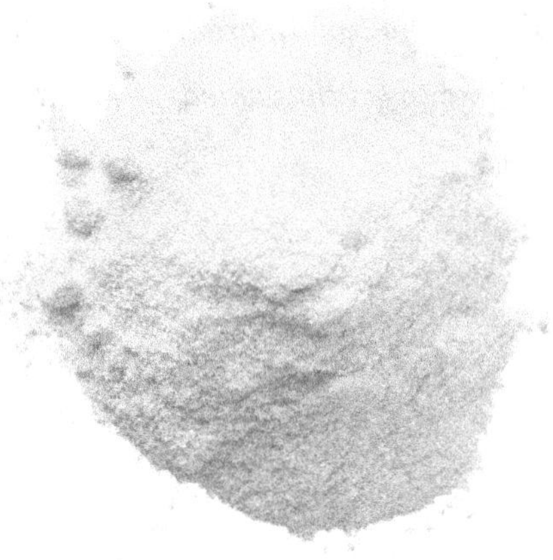

Sulphur

The Sulphur Case

A three year old child

He has been sick since he was born. At birth he already had patches of eczema all over the body.

He's caught a cold for the first time a month after birth. It happened in the first cold days in early autumn, and the heating in city wasn't on yet. That is when he's got the first bronchitis, and after that he was getting bronchitis practically every month, so he was ill almost all the time. He was getting Berodual (generic fenoterol and ipratropium bromide, anticholinergic) all the time, because he was constantly in risk of suffocation.

He is feeling better when we go to the seaside, but every time he gets bronchitis at the last night of our stay. Last time he's got so cyanotic that he was half living, half dead. He was kicking and screaming on the plane. When we came to the hospital, we were told he was in the first stage of pneumonia. We were in hospital for ten days. Now he is taking Flixotid (genericfluticasone propionate, corticosteroid) one inhalation twice a day and Aerius (generic desloratadine, antihistaminic).

He coughs at night, with coughing up thick mucus. It sounds like his lungs will tear apart of coughing. He's also felt pain in left ear. He sweats a lot. His adenoid was surgically removed, but he didn't get any better.

We also have problems with feeding him, because he is allergic to milk, eggs and peanuts. He drinks only rise milk since he was born. Even he knows which kinds of food are not allowed to him. It's a problem on birthday's parties, because everyone is eating and he can't...

He is lively and short tempered by nature, but he can be delightful, friendly, sweet and talkative. Everybody likes him very much. He has a rash on the skin that looks like wheat grits. He is warm-blooded and likes to take off his clothes. His eyes are often getting crusty.

No one in his family has had similar difficulties, except for his father who used to have chronic bronchitis when he was a child, but not as frequent or as early in life… His uncle also had some respiratory difficulties, but no one on my side of the family.

Based on the child's appearance, constitution, temper, behavior, warm bloodedness, being prone to sweating, mostly left sided diseases and in the way rush on his skin looked, we have decided to give the patient homeopathic remedy,

Rp. Sulphur C30

We have also instructed his mother what to do if he gets a high fever...

Follow-up after one week

We have reduced using the inhaler to a minimum right after the remedy was given. He feels great! He didn't have any kind of difficulties. We have given him food that you have told us to and nothing has happened to him!!! He didn't get a rash. He is so happy! For the first time in his life he can eat what other children can… We are all very happy because of that.

only a week has passed,

℞. Watch and wait

Follow-up after one week

We have completely stopped using the inhaler. He breathes very well. He's got a runny nose. He sneezes and then he has a thick, white, falling snot. He's got some reddish spots all over his body, and a rash that looks like wheat grits on his chest.

He eats all kinds of food and he's got a good appetite. He likes yoghurt most of all.

Everything is going well, so we've decided to repeat the remedy in higher potency.

℞. Sulphur C200

Follow-up after twelve days

We went to the swimming pool. He's got big red spots above the eye, on the neck, scapula, like he had ones when he ate peanuts.

He used to have that sun allergy before, just like his father. It also happened from walnuts once and then had a rash all over his body, just like when he eats peanuts. Then he was given Urbason (generic methylprednisolone, corticosteroid).

This time, at the swimming pool, that red rush was spreading all over his body, but breathing was fine all the time. I got frightened, because the hospital was far away and it was Sunday. Anyway, the rash began to fade, all by itself and half an hour later it disappeared completely, without taking any kind of allopathic medications.

His breathing was fine all the time, he didn't cough, he had a good appetite, he could eat anything and he wasn't taking any medications. He is as healthy as you can only wish.

Since the child's breathing is fine, he can eat anything, he has a good appetite, he is in a good mood and sleeps well, we've decided to,

Rp. Watch and wait

Follow-up after one month

He feels fine and everything is all right. Some kind of redness appeared in the inner corners of his eyes for the last few days. We didn't notice anything else.

Everything is great. His breathing is fine and he eats like a horse!

Everything is going as well as expected, because children have a strong vital force.

Rp. Watch and wait

Follow-up after three days

Today he vomited everything he ate. First he had a runny nose yesterday, then coughing started, then he had a difficulty breathing and in the evening he got a fever... We were using cold applications according to your instructions, he started sweating and the fever dropped... He was expectorating thick mucus. His appetite was worse. He didn't eat, because he vomited everything because of that thick mucus. Other than that he is in a good mood. His stool is soft. His tongue is red, like a raspberry. He has an allergic reaction in the face and back from the sun...

The high fever points out a good immunological response! We'll repeat the remedy in the same potency.

Rp. Sulph c200

Follow-up after ten days

Yesterday we arrived from the seaside. Everything was fine. We were afraid of the trip back home, because we use to end up in hospital every time , we were coming back from the seaside, using Urbason. This time everything went great!

After the last remedy we went to the seaside. his nose

was a little runny, with sneezing and thick greenish snots, but soon it became a watery discharge.

He had diarrhea one day, probably because he swallowed some sea water.

He had a rash on his thighs, neck and the scalp. It was itching, especially when he was sweating.

His reaction to the remedy is great. He's got thick, green nose discharge, the disorder from the lungs came out to the surface, on the skin. He generally feels great, so

Rp. Watch and wait

Follow-up after three weeks

Everything is great!

His breathing is fine and he doesn't cough. He eats everything. He likes milk, cheese and yoghurt the most.

He have become more reasonable, relaxed and calmer. We are all satisfied.

Everything is fine.

Rp. Watch and wait

Follow-up after one month

He went to the seaside again and on his way back he went to the mountains. Everything was fine.

Rp. Watch and wait

Follow-up in two months, or earlier if necessary. We have also instructed the mother how to recognize the symptoms that would indicate the time to come back and repeat the remedy.

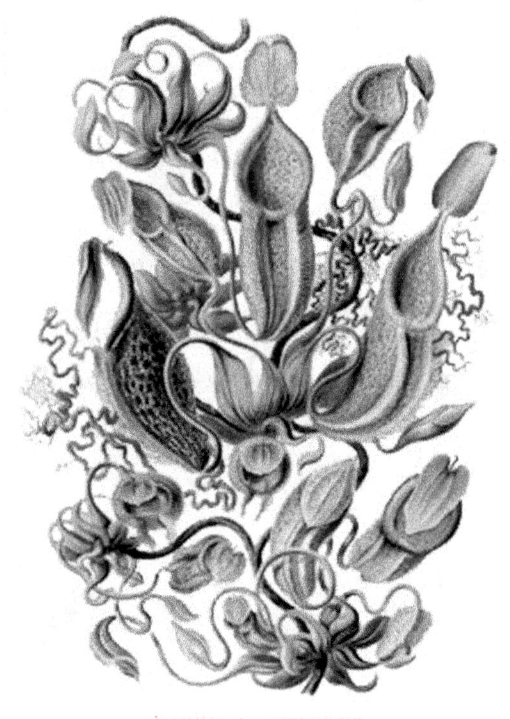

Drosera
Rotundifolia

The Drosera Case

A thirty year old woman, clerk

I came because of my gynecological issues. I haven't heard of that kind of medicine before. I was sent by my gynecologist. My diagnosis is Erosio cervicis planocellulare (CIN - Cervical intraepithelial neoplasia), and I'm HPV (Human papillomavirus) positive. I haven't had any significant health conditions before this. I have two children. A nine year old boy and a six year old girl. My period is regular. I have a severe backache during PMS, so sometimes I can't bend forward.

I'm stressed out and under pressure at work, because my position is somewhere in-between. I'm neither an ordinary clerk, nor high ranking. I can't be productive without some necessary changes in the business policy in my firm, on which I have no influence, and on the other hand I'm under constant pressure for better results from the higher ranks… My husband is at home with the kids. He cooks and works in his home office, while I am at work all day long. I arrive home late, around 5 p.m. I argue a lot with my colleagues at work… I get nervous, light a cigarette and try to cool down. Sometimes some of us at work don't speak for days, after arguing.

Somehow I manage to stay calmer than the others. They are so presumptuous and envious. One of them has accused me of lying. One of them has a "difficult personality", so once she told me: "You walk all over me." Sometimes I have a stomach ache, so I feel some kind of pressure and spasm. I feel the acid reflux and stinging. I have a pure circulation, cold hands and feet. I'm chilly. I use a duvet even in the summer. I've got small pimples under my eyes, and they used to appear on my forehead. My skin and hair are greasy. I regularly go to the beauty salon.

I love the sea, and it makes me feel good. I can swim for a long time.I love tweezing my eyebrows! It makes me calm and relaxed. It makes me feel good, because I'm aiming something!

I have a hypertrophic tissue in the region of the thyroid gland, and hormone levels are elevated. I usually have low blood pressure and the iron level in blood is also inadequate.

I have had vitiligo for 18 years. There is a white spot on my face, arm pit, inguinal region, hip, chest, arms and right elbow. In the summer these spots used to get burned and desquamate, like lichen. It gets burned, red, in the sun, and then back to white.

When I was a child I used to have problems with my lungs, bronchitis and cough. I even had a biopsy of the lung. I don't remember exactly how it went, only that they said that my lungs were not resistant to tuberculosis, because vaccines couldn't have any effect.

Based on the impression of an arrogant, haughty, strong personality, talkative, loud, stomach problems, with a history of respiratory conditions in her childhood, we have decided to give a remedy of tubercular miasmas.

Rp. Drosera rotundifolia C200

Follow-up after one month

The first day after the remedy I had a terrible headache, with vomiting. I got better very fast, in one day.

We went to the seaside. It was beautiful. I was sleeping on the beach, even for two hours, like a baby. I was perfectly relaxed, like a long time ago.

My vitiligo has got smaller on the left hand! Pigmentation has started appearing on the white spots…

Pimples have appeared on my face, with the biggest one on the chin, that looked like it's hormonal.

I didn't get into any conflicts at work.

The first day after the remedy there was an aggravation followed by a headache and vomiting, and that was cleansing of the organism.

Then a good mental state followed, and changes are expected on all other levels. Pigmentation started to appear in the vitiligo white spots. Everything is going well, so we' ve decided to,

Rp. Watch and wait

Follow-up after one month

My health is fine. There is some reorganizing going on at work. It's a very hard period. Many of us will be fired. I couldn't sleep for two nights because of the problems at work.

I'm less nervous than I was before the treatment, but I still feel uneasy. Pimples are still appearing on my face, especially on the forehead and cheeks…

There is a new order and harmony in the patient's organism, as well as in her life. The suppressed disorders are getting out on the skin, in the form of pimples.

Rp. Drosera rotundifolia C200

Follow-up after one month

I've decided to have a third child. The situation at home is good, and I'm getting along with my husband well.

At work we are still in the process of reorganizing and

firing. I'm less stressed – what happens, happens. I don't feel any pain in the stomach anymore. The pimples are slowly disappearing…

The patient looks self-assured and calm. Everything is going well, so we've decided to

Rp. Watch and wait

Follow-up after two months

I have been at the gynecologist. I'm pregnant! My pap test result came back normal!!!

At work of us six female employees, four are pregnant… I feel fine. I don't feel any kind of unease… Thyroid hormone T4 results are better than they used to be. All of my test results are fine…

The patient's state is excellent. Not only is her cervix healed, but as a proof of her good general health she's got pregnant again.

The pregnancy can also protect her from being fired at

work. The homeopathic treatment helped our patient to harmonize her health, and by doing so, all other aspects of her life, too.

Rp. Watch and wait

Follow-up when necessary. The patient is advised to come before her delivery for instructions, and a set of homeopathic remedies...

This book may help people to realize that there is a light, swift and gentle method of healing, that leads to a state of harmony, peace and well-being, for the patient as well as his family and others around him or her, because the change in one causes changes on the whole.

If you are seeking prosperity, knowledge and truth, homeopathy is the method of healing that can make it possible and opens the path to self-realization.

We have tried to show this art in its elegant, beautiful, simple and true form. When the case is shown in its very essence, the homeopathic treatment looks simple and easy, but it's the result of years of painstaking devoted work of the homeopathic practitioner. The cases described here are not supposed to be used as a guide how to prescribe these particular remedies, because this is just the essence, an overview of case taking, but to show some of the ways in which homeopathy has changed real lives for the better.

I wish to express my gratitude to everyone who has helped in the creation of this book. First to my spiritual teachers, as well as to the people who gave me their trust and where willing to work on themselves and change, and by doing so, to change the world a bit for the better.

I wish to express my gratitude to all the people who've supported me selflessly, to make it possible for this book to see its dawn, light of the new sunrise.

I wish to express my gratitude to the one who deserves to be thanked!

THANK YOU

www.ingramcontent.com/pod-product-compliance
Lightning Source LLC
Chambersburg PA
CBHW060502280326
41933CB00014B/2831

* 9 7 8 8 6 9 1 4 2 6 3 2 3 *